Distribution, publication, and copying in any form are prohibited and subject to damages.

# TEN HYPNOSES

Copying, publishing, and sharing with third parties are only permitted with the written consent of the author. Please observe the notes on copyright and usage.

Distribution, publication, and copying in any form are prohibited and subject to damages.

Copying, publishing, and sharing with third parties are only permitted with the written consent of the author. Please observe the notes on copyright and usage.

Distribution, publication, and copying in any form are prohibited and subject to damages.

Ingo Michael Simon

# TEN HYPNOSES

22

S̲e̲l̲f̲-A̲w̲a̲r̲e̲n̲e̲s̲s̲ ̲a̲n̲d̲ ̲S̲e̲l̲f̲-L̲o̲v̲e̲

Copying, publishing, and sharing with third parties are only permitted with the written consent of the author. Please observe the notes on copyright and usage.

Distribution, publication, and copying in any form are prohibited and subject to damages.

© 2024 Ingo Michael Simon
All rights reserved.
Independently published
www.ingosimon.com

Important Notes for Urgent Attention:
The contents of this book are based on the practical experiences of the author with hypnosis applications and psychotherapy in a trance state. Although the author has strived for the utmost care, errors or misunderstandings in the presentation cannot be completely excluded. Therapeutic work with people and the application of hypnosis are solely the responsibility of the hypnotist. It cannot be ruled out that parts of this book may be misunderstood or that the application of a presented procedure may cause an undesirable reaction in the client. The author also assumes no co-responsibility if work with a client is carried out with reference to the statements in this book.

The Author:
Ingo Michael Simon studied psychology and education and is a hypnotherapist with practices in southwestern Germany and Switzerland. With the help of hypnosis-supported psychotherapy, he primarily treats people with persistent psychological conditions. His practice focuses on anxiety disorders, pathological compulsions, and psychosomatic illnesses. His therapeutic offerings mainly include classical and modern hypnosis applications and the dreamland therapy he developed himself.

Copying, publishing, and sharing with third parties are only permitted with the written consent of the author. Please observe the notes on copyright and usage.

## Notes on Copyright and Usage

Copying, publishing, and sharing with third parties is prohibited and only permitted with the written consent of the author. Please observe the following copyright and usage guidelines.

This work has been carefully crafted and created to the best of the author's knowledge and personal experience. It comprises text templates and application guidelines for professional hypnosis sessions. The author is a licensed psychotherapist with extensive experience in psychotherapy, coaching, and personal training using hypnotic techniques and methods. Nevertheless, the author and the publisher assume no liability for the accuracy of information, instructions, and advice, nor for any typographical errors. The author and publisher accept no responsibility or liability for the application of these texts and recommendations with clients or patients, nor for any potential consequences or unexpected reactions. It is expressly noted that the application of therapeutic and advisory techniques and formulations lies solely and entirely within the responsibility of the practitioner. This also applies to adherence to the boundaries of legally regulated medical and therapeutic practices. The fact that a book containing action proposals is freely available for sale does not imply that its application with clients or patients is permitted for everyone.

Distribution, publication, and copying in any form are prohibited and subject to damages.

Copying, publishing, and sharing with third parties are only permitted with the written consent of the author. Please observe the notes on copyright and usage.

Distribution, publication, and copying in any form are prohibited and subject to damages.

## Table of Contents

Introduction ........................................................................................................ 1

Hypnosis 1 .......................................................................................................... 1

Hypnosis 2 .......................................................................................................... 1

Hypnosis 3 .......................................................................................................... 1

Hypnosis 4 .......................................................................................................... 1

Hypnosis 5 .......................................................................................................... 1

Hypnosis 6 .......................................................................................................... 1

Hypnosis 7 .......................................................................................................... 1

Hypnosis 8 .......................................................................................................... 1

Hypnosis 9 .......................................................................................................... 1

Hypnosis 10 ........................................................................................................ 1

Overview of All Titles in the Series "Ten Hypnoses" ......................................... 1

Copying, publishing, and sharing with third parties are only permitted with the written consent of the author. Please observe the notes on copyright and usage.

Distribution, publication, and copying in any form are prohibited and subject to damages.

Copying, publishing, and sharing with third parties are only permitted with the written consent of the author. Please observe the notes on copyright and usage.

# Introduction

The series "Ten Hypnoses" is very well known in Germany, Austria, and Switzerland as a collection of texts for therapeutic work and is used by numerous psychotherapeutic practices, doctors, therapists, coaches, and other helping professionals. I am pleased to now be able to offer these texts in other countries as well.

Most therapists have their own methods for inducing and deepening trance as well as for exiting trance. Therefore, I have focused on the main part of the hypnosis. The texts in this book can be integrated as the main part into any hypnosis process.

The texts in this collection use various hypnosis techniques. I will not explain these in detail, as I assume that users have the appropriate training. It is also not necessary to understand the exact structure or functioning of the different parts. The texts can simply be read aloud, and they will have their effect.

Decide for yourself which text best suits your client or patient at any given time. You can also combine passages from different texts. It is not about using all ten hypnoses in sequence. It is a selection of possibilities.

I want to emphasize that books cannot replace therapy. Psychotherapy or other therapeutic treatments involve much more. A careful diagnosis is the necessary basis for deciding on the use of methods, including whether hypnosis or one of my texts should be used. Even in this case, preparatory discussions, follow-up discussions during the session, and of course, a therapeutic concept for the sequence of sessions and the content approaches are essential parts of therapy. This cannot and should not be achieved with a collection of texts.

In any case, I wish you much success in your work and I am pleased if my text templates can contribute in a small way.

*Ingo Michael Simon*

Distribution, publication, and copying in any form are prohibited and subject to damages.

Copying, publishing, and sharing with third parties are only permitted with the written consent of the author. Please observe the notes on copyright and usage.

# Hypnosis 1

Setting Goals and Strengthening Willpower

Today, you have decided to experience a unique strength within yourself... Today, you will feel that you are truly valuable and good... Today, you can find and intensify the feeling of self-respect... and from this, draw hope and trust... trust in life and above all, trust in yourself... You are fully focusing your strength to feel deeper within yourself and to let your gaze go deeper into your inner center, because that is where the source of your mindfulness lies... mindfulness from you for you... mindfulness from you for you...

It's truly amazing how quickly you find and experience your self-awareness today, starting right now... This step is special for you, because you are becoming the center of your life at this moment, for nothing and no one is more important than yourself right now... This moment is just for you... only for you...

## Aligning Thoughts

This is the special thought that fills you... this one thought that tells you... I am aware of myself and I respect myself because I am a valuable person... and whenever you think it consciously, when you formulate it in your mind, it feels right and good... I am aware of myself and I respect myself because I am a valuable person... This is the thought of this moment... it is a thought that becomes more natural and more self-evident... It is a thought that guides and supports you... and this thought also helps you to deal with yourself mindfully and carefully... to take yourself seriously and importantly... This thought helps you to really feel that you are valuable... and that the moment is valuable when you are fully with yourself... just like now... Your self-acceptance becomes a feeling of self-love...

## Somatic Alignment (Body Suggestion)

Your body can feel the state of inner calm at this moment and you can clearly sense this feeling... You feel inside yourself and can feel this deep relaxation you are now in... This state allows your feeling to be present and to become more mindful and to accept and like yourself more as you are... to like yourself exactly as you are... Your body helps you because it shows you with its relaxation that inner acceptance is working, that it really succeeds to become one with your own feeling... because accepting yourself means becoming one with your own feeling... this is what you achieve and you can see and feel it in the relaxation of your body... You can feel it... your calm helps you...

Emotional Alignment (Feeling Suggestion)

You go even deeper into your feelings and you are completely there... in your inner center, where all your feelings are... and at this moment a special feeling arises... the feeling of self-love... initially as a feeling that you are truly valuable and important... and with every breath, this feeling becomes more beautiful and intense... with every breath you feel that the feeling of self-respect becomes clearer... so clear that you can already find yourself really good... that you can accept yourself as you are... and finally, that you can love yourself... perhaps you can already feel it clearly at this second or you will feel it clearly in a few moments... after a few breaths... You succeed in loving yourself more... you succeed here and now... at this moment... Your self-respect becomes self-love... Now... Your self-respect becomes self-love... Now...

### Behavioral Alignment

You are now changing your behavior towards yourself... You decide to hold onto your mindfulness and to always feel that it is there and growing... You decide to take better care of yourself... to respect your feelings more and to feel what you truly feel... You firmly decide to spend a daily time of contemplation just with yourself... entirely in your feeling... and to accept and like yourself... to love yourself... a daily time of stillness becomes daily self-love... Love from you for you... Love from you for you...

### Outlook and Vision

You think about how it will be in your everyday life with your new self-love... You imagine in inner images and thoughts how it will be when you go into the day with this new feeling of self-awareness... You imagine how beautiful it will be because you will listen more and more to what your feeling tells you... because you will trust more and more that your deep feelings are good and right and guide you... You will no longer hand over the decisions of your life... You will decide for yourself, because you know you can rely on yourself and on your feelings...

## Summary

The time has come and it can no longer be otherwise than to put yourself completely in the center of your mindfulness... to put yourself in the focus of your care and attention... You have decided and even better: You have done it today, you have fully embraced this thought that tells you... I am aware of myself and I respect myself because I am a valuable person... This thought is now your new fundamental attitude... With this thought, which imprints itself on your body feeling and thus becomes a matter of course, you start each day... I am aware of myself and I respect myself because I am a valuable person...

# Hypnosis 2

## Preparation

You know self-doubt and self-alienation... You have experienced it yourself... In the stress and burdens of life, you have distanced yourself from yourself and then you were like separated from yourself... You tried to change that... tried to think and feel differently... Sometimes it may have even succeeded, but then self-doubt returned... But that is good news, because you have also repeatedly succeeded in turning towards yourself mindfully and lovingly... So it succeeds today as well... Today you achieve a real self-approach and a true connection to yourself... Today you achieve a lasting connection... Today you achieve a lasting renewal... and then a new feeling of mindfulness and turning towards yourself arises... For this, you first go within and meet yourself... Today, you go deep into your feeling... deeper than usual... Today, your gaze turns inward completely, and with your gaze, your thoughts turn inward... and with your thoughts, your feelings turn inward... because that is where the truly new begins... within yourself... in your deep feeling... in your emotions, which are different from what you might have thought... So let's take this step... the first and decisive step of self-love...

## Self-Acceptance

Accept the past time of self-alienation and distance from yourself... because all of it is part of you and your personal history...

{about 5-10 seconds of silence}

Accept the past time of self-alienation and distance from yourself... because that way you can process your past and be close to yourself again...

{about 5-10 seconds of silence}

Accept the past time of self-alienation and distance from yourself... because that way you can let go of self-doubt right now and be free...

{about 5-10 seconds of silence}

Accept the past time of self-alienation and distance from yourself... because that way you can create a new and good feeling of life...

{about 5-10 seconds of silence}

Accept the past time of self-alienation and distance from yourself... because that way you find your way back to yourself, to your self-love...

{about 5-10 seconds of silence}

Self-Forgiveness

Forgive yourself for not taking care of your feelings...

because you know you have never acted culpably...

{about 5-10 seconds of silence}

Forgive yourself for not taking care of your feelings...

because now you are truly ready to be one with yourself again...

{about 5-10 seconds of silence}

Forgive yourself for not taking care of your feelings...

because now you are truly ready to look forward...

{about 5-10 seconds of silence}

Forgive yourself for not taking care of your feelings...

because now you are truly ready to fully accept yourself...

{about 5-10 seconds of silence}

Forgive yourself for not taking care of your feelings...

because now you are truly ready to be yourself...

{about 5-10 seconds of silence}

Self-Love

Engage with your sensations and feelings and feel yourself... with the certainty that you really want to...

{about 5-10 seconds of silence}

Engage with your sensations and feelings and feel yourself... with the certainty that you really can...

{about 5-10 seconds of silence}

Engage with your sensations and feelings and feel yourself... with the certainty that you are truly worth being loved...

{about 5-10 seconds of silence}

Engage with your sensations and feelings and feel yourself... with the certainty that self-love accompanies you vibrantly...

{about 5-10 seconds of silence}

Engage with your sensations and feelings and feel yourself... with the certainty that your self-love is real and honest...

{about 5-10 seconds of silence}

# Hypnosis 3

Anchor Technique (Perihypnotic Anchor)

*An anchor (or trigger) is a stimulus that is intended to evoke a specific feeling or awaken a particular thought. It is a signal perceived by the client, initiating an internal process. The established anchor then replaces the suggestion. In everyday life, a client can use an anchor to induce or establish a desired state even without a trance state. Numerous stimuli can serve as anchors/triggers. I work with the following possibilities, which I also use in the series "Ten Hypnoses": Body anchors (closing the hand, pressing the thumb pad...), visual anchors (symbols, word cards...), acoustic anchors (signal noises like phone ringing, melodies...), olfactory anchors (scent oils...), tactile anchors (comfort stones, talismans...). I also distinguish between perihypnotic and posthypnotic anchors. Perihypnotic anchors are those primarily used during hypnosis by the therapist to set up the anchor and then trigger it repeatedly to complement suggestions and visualizations. Posthypnotic anchors are mainly set up for the time after the session so that the client can help themselves with them.*

### Preparing the Anchor Technique

Today we are working with a very special scent... with a technique that makes it much easier for you to accept yourself and even find yourself good... soon to even love yourself... To make this possible, you will learn about the scent of self-love today... whenever you can perceive it, you will remember deep inside that you may and want to accept yourself...

[Prepare a bottle with a pleasant scent oil. You need to be able to open and close it. It should be a somewhat intrusive scent that the client has not already used. For example, if the client loves vanilla, this scent is already strongly emotionally associated, as well as perfume. It works best if it is a "new" scent that we suggestively charge with the hypnosis. However, it does not have to be an unknown scent. It should just not be one regularly used by the client.]

### Creating the Desired Emotional State

Now, first and foremost, deep calm is important... because in deep calm and relaxation, it is much easier to accept yourself... to be relaxed and to deal with yourself in a relaxed manner... for this, you can now relax even deeper and feel how good deep relaxation actually feels... how easy it can be to be internally calm... and in calmness to accept yourself... very good... You relax... You can do it... It is going very well... You just let go... You feel a deep and pleasant relaxation in you... and you have the desire to go even deeper into this beautiful relaxation... deeply relaxed...

Setting Up the Anchor

Now in pleasant relaxation, you can meet yourself with calmness, let go of all criticism, and accept yourself... It is much easier now than usual... You accept yourself at this moment... The more clearly you can feel the relaxation now, the better you can accept yourself... Feel the relaxation and accept yourself... Now... Now it works... You can feel calm... [Open the bottle and bring it to the client's nose]... You can accept yourself... [Take the bottle away and close it]... This is a special step because you can actually do it... [Open the bottle and bring it to the client's nose]... You can accept yourself... [Take the bottle away and close it]... Perhaps you already imagine how nice it would be if you could always feel calm... [Open the bottle and bring it to the client's nose]... and accept yourself at the same time... [Take the bottle away and close it]... Calm and accept yourself at the same time... [Open the bottle and bring it to the client's nose]... You can accept yourself... [Take the bottle away and close it]...

[The chosen scent has now become an anchor. Each further presentation of the scent awakens or emphasizes this feeling again. The client can then focus on their thoughts and wishes and always receive an impulse to feel relaxation and self-acceptance simultaneously. As a perihypnotic anchor, the chosen scent can be used in subsequent sessions without needing to be set up again.]

Using the Anchor

Think again about your self-image... consider how you can see yourself and how you can manage to find yourself good... [Open the bottle and bring it to the client's nose]... It has changed because you can now accept yourself better... [Take the bottle away and close it]... Often, you had self-doubt and struggled with yourself, unable to allow yourself to truly accept yourself... perhaps thinking that it would only succeed over time... [Open the bottle and bring it to the client's nose]... That was in the past... [Take the bottle away and close it]... Now it is different... now you can let go of self-criticism much better... simply accept yourself as you are... It succeeds because you remain calm and considerate with yourself... [Open the bottle and bring it to the client's nose]... You can accept yourself... [Take the bottle away and close it]...

Reinforcement (Posthypnotic Suggestion)

It is truly amazing how quickly you have managed to initiate an important change... to accept yourself much better than before... That is good... You have learned that you can indeed adjust yourself if you are open... open to your perceptions... to the scent... and open to your self-awareness... and whenever you inhale this scent... when you can perceive it... [Open the bottle and bring it to the client's nose]... it reminds you that you can and may love yourself... [Take the bottle away and close it]... Today and every day of your life...

# Hypnosis 4

Anchor Technique (Posthypnotic Anchor)

*An anchor (or trigger) is a stimulus that is intended to evoke a specific feeling or awaken a particular thought. It is a signal perceived by the client, initiating an internal process. The established anchor then replaces the suggestion. In everyday life, a client can use an anchor to induce or establish a desired state even without a trance state. Numerous stimuli can serve as anchors/triggers. I work with the following possibilities, which I also use in the series "Ten Hypnoses": Body anchors (closing the hand, pressing the thumb pad...), visual anchors (symbols, word cards...), acoustic anchors (signal noises like phone ringing, melodies...), olfactory anchors (scent oils...), tactile anchors (comfort stones, talismans...). I also distinguish between perihypnotic and posthypnotic anchors. Perihypnotic anchors are those primarily used during hypnosis by the therapist to set up the anchor and then trigger it repeatedly to complement suggestions and visualizations. Posthypnotic* anchors are mainly set up for the time after the session so that the client can help themselves with them.

### Preparing the Anchor Technique

Today we are working with a special method... with a ritual that can help you to accept yourself much better... to accept yourself repeatedly... to forgive yourself when you reproach yourself... We call this a hypnosis anchor... Once this anchor is set up, it works always and everywhere... and setting up the anchor is simple... I will show you how it works and help you... You can then use the anchor anytime and anywhere to connect with yourself... to accept yourself and even to love yourself... For this, later when I prompt you, place both hands crossed over your chest so that you can feel the warmth of your palms on your body...

### Creating the Desired Emotional State

Now, first and foremost, it's about a very pleasant and deep relaxation... because in truly deep and pleasant relaxation, you can feel yourself with all your feelings much better... and that's what it's about... feeling your own feelings as they are... whether pleasant or unpleasant... Accepting yourself means feeling what is really there and accepting it... This then frees you from painful feelings, because only when they are allowed to be, can they also pass... It is the struggle against painful feelings that causes them to stay... Follow the rhythm of your breathing and come to rest... it happens naturally if you just focus on the flow of your breath and imagine it becoming calmer... It gets quieter and quieter outside and inside... quieter and quieter inside you... and you come closer and closer to your inner center... come close to your feelings... and closer and closer... You rest within yourself and feel yourself... feel the connection to yourself... and imagine thoughts and feelings flowing into each other like two liquids... and becoming one... Thoughts and feelings become one...

Setting Up the Anchor

You speak in your mind the sentence: I am connected with myself... and as you do, your feelings and thoughts flow even more into each other and become one... You can feel how you come closer to yourself with this... Now it is much easier to say: I accept myself... I accept myself... Now, place both arms crossed over your chest and place the palms on your body...

[Wait until the client has placed their hands on their chest as prompted. If they do not follow the prompt immediately, which is rare, wait a few seconds and then prompt again... Now we want to set up the important anchor for you, place your arms crossed over your body and touch your chest with your palms...]

...Good, now feel your hands on your body... Feel the connection to your warmth... Warmth from you for you... Connection from you to you... Your body has already understood that the contact of your hands to your body is a signal for inner, emotional self-connection... a step of self-acceptance... and if you want to feel the connection to yourself even deeper now, press your hands a little firmer on your body... feeling more warmth and equally more connection to yourself... good... very good... Your anchor works... Now release the pressure... very slowly, because then you can best feel that the feeling of connection to yourself remains... Once your anchor is triggered, once you place your hands on your body like now, your whole body, your whole organism, goes into the feeling of self-connection and stays there for as long as possible... Take your hands completely off your body and feel that this feeling of connection indeed remains... and if you want to strengthen this feeling, place your hands crossed on your chest again, do it now and feel the connection and closeness even more...

### Reinforcement (Posthypnotic Suggestion)

Good... You have already done everything you need... have successfully set up the anchor and can use it anytime from now on... Whenever you feel the need to connect with yourself more, simply place your hands on your body and immediately feel the deeper connection... immediately connect with yourself and can accept yourself... You can make it a daily practice... In a moment of contemplation and calm, do it daily just as you did here today... You place your arms as your anchor on your body and can accept yourself... can endure and bear yourself... can love yourself... You can love yourself... You managed it here and today... You can do it every day anew and again...

# Hypnosis 5

### Goal Setting and Preparation

You want to take better care of yourself... because you feel it is time to finally do that... not just be there for others, but entirely for yourself... because now you are the one who needs your help the most... You need your mindfulness and affection... You want to feel your own love... Surely, you have heard that only those who are there for themselves can truly be there for others... and that is really true... You have already managed to put yourself aside and be there for others... but you have become unhappy in the process... have lost strength... have lost yourself... but now you are finding yourself again... coming back to yourself, to be fully there for yourself... with mindfulness and love... with self-mindfulness and self-love...

### Perspective Change

Imagine you could carry your self-regard with you like a ball... a big light ball, filled with mindfulness and calm... with self-love... Imagine it in a color of your choice... maybe it should be a colorful, bright ball... with a beautiful pattern... Imagine it... so big that you can carry it well... that you can tuck it under your arm and carry it with you because it is very light... and if you hold it against the sun, it shines even more and you can feel the feeling in it and use it for yourself... with a look at the sun, you feel the self-love that you carry with you and in you... like a ball that you always hold on to... This ball of self-love has always existed, but you have left it lying... so you often could not feel affection for yourself... could not handle yourself mindfully... had to search for the ball first... But now you take it with you... hold it, tuck it under your arm and imagine meeting other people while carrying your self-love with you... holding it firmly...

Re-evaluating Own Experiences

You now dive into your memories again and think of a situation in which you could not accept yourself at all... Imagine the situation again and imagine you had accepted yourself... with all the feelings you had... maybe you could have acted differently, but imagine you had accepted yourself with your feelings... You would have carried the ball with you, only one hand free for others... only one hand to help, because one would have held this ball... Probably you could have helped less... could not have packed so firmly for others... but you could not have neglected yourself either, because you would have had the ball of self-mindfulness with you... a balanced relationship between being there for others and for yourself... maybe your help would have taken longer... maybe it would have been harder with only one free hand to help... You would have needed a break sooner... but you would have always been with yourself too... But you mostly thought you had to put your ball aside and only pick it up again when everything else was done... So sometimes in the hustle of time and among all the demands you wanted to fulfill, you forgot to pick up your ball again... or you simply couldn't manage it anymore...

Action Change

Imagine wanting to help a person carry a heavy jug of water... a jug with two handles... earlier you might have carried it alone to relieve this person... but now that is not possible, because you only have one hand free... but that is good... that is very good... because this person also has only one hand free... They carry their own ball like you... Imagine now how you both can carry the jug together... each only with one hand and with joint strength... and each carries their own self-mindfulness and self-love... Imagine it as a picture... and imagine that you can always help this way... help but also be with yourself... help others and help yourself... So you can be there for others even better because your strength also remains with you and for you... it is just a picture... an imagination... but any imagination can become truth if you are ready for it... and this picture can help you more and more to focus on respecting and loving yourself... more and more... it is as simple as carrying a ball... just as simple as carrying a ball...

Reinforcement (Posthypnotic Suggestion)

You now feel the inner calm and relaxation... You feel and know that you can and may always carry your self-respect and self-love with you... You feel and know that you do not have to neglect yourself to help others... So you start each day with the imagination of picking up a big light ball and carrying it with you all day... and with it always carrying self-respect and self-love with you and making sure to always hold them... just like a ball when carrying the jug together...

# Hypnosis 6

### Goal Setting and Preparation

For a long time, you have had the wish to be able to accept yourself better... to be one with yourself and then be able to feel self-love again... maybe even to feel this feeling properly for the first time... You have already taken an important first step because you are here, which is only possible because you matter to yourself... because you do like yourself and want to help yourself... So you can take further steps, take better and deeper care of yourself... and feel that you are always close to yourself, even when you couldn't grasp it well, you were connected to yourself... But you want and can feel it... with mindfulness and turning towards yourself...

### Perspective Change

You often had little time for yourself because you had to take care of so many people and things... thought of yourself too late... maybe you thought it had to be that way... but today you can do it differently... Here and today, you do not have to take care of anyone else but yourself... Now is the time just for you and your feeling... now you can allow yourself to be close to yourself... to perceive yourself... to accept yourself... and respect yourself... now you can open up to yourself... like a closed bud opening in the light and warmth of the sun... Your gaze turns more and more towards yourself... now it is easier because now there is nothing to accomplish... now you have no duties... maybe only the duty to take care of yourself... a beautiful and peaceful duty that protects you and places you in the center because that is where you belong... in the center of your life... like a closed bud that you hold in your hands and hide there safely...

Re-evaluating Own Experiences

Sometimes you thought you were in your own way... that you were preventing yourself from meeting yourself mindfully and lovingly... but like the bud that is closed and yet beautiful inside and ready to bloom, so was this part of you alive... just protected and withdrawn... like a closed bud or bud that you hide safely in your hand so it cannot break... so you have preserved and protected this part of you... until the right time comes to open this inner bud now... to allow the inner blooming... and maybe this right moment is just now... this moment that counts... the right time to bloom...

Action Change

The time has come... the time is ripe... It is time to bloom... to free yourself and open up like a radiant flower... in all its colorful splendor and beauty... Imagine the sun shining above you... It warms you and envelops your whole body in a warming cloak... and in your hands, hidden, you hold a closed bud... the bud of your self-love... it is in you... like a bud waiting to bloom... You hold it in your hands... and the sun warms your hands pleasantly... Then you prepare to open the inner bud of self-love... You imagine that it actually succeeds because you want it so... because you really want to accept and love yourself... today as much as possible and tomorrow even more... You open your hands and look at the closed bud lying in them... the bud of your self-love... It is enclosed with green leaves... and the sunlight, the warming rays shine on this bud... these warming rays come from within you... they are the rays of mindfulness that shine when you turn towards yourself... and exactly that you have already done... You have turned towards... towards yourself and placed yourself at the center of your efforts... this effort for yourself is pure mindfulness... your mindfulness for you... from you for you... and this mindfulness shines within you and warms the bud like the summer sun in the morning... and slowly, step by step, the bud opens in your hand... slowly, the feeling of love unfolds in your own hand... Love from you for you... your self-love... it opens and unfolds more and more... more and more... Self-love unfolds now... in the sunlight of your mindfulness... The bud opens and shines in your favorite colors... it blooms before your inner eye in the most beautiful colors you can imagine... until it fully opens and fully unfolds and stretches towards the warmth and light... The feeling of self-love rises within you and unfolds like the bud in the sunlight...

Reinforcement (Posthypnotic Suggestion)

You imagine that it can be good to feel the feeling of self-love every day... to let it rise from your inner center... to unfold self-love like the bud in the sunlight... You make the connection clear again... Mindfulness is like sunlight... and self-love like a closed bud that wants to unfold... with a moment of mindfulness towards yourself, the warming sunlight meets the bud of self-love, which immediately unfolds... every day this can happen... with just a moment of self-mindfulness, which you succeed as well as today... and self-love unfolds... You simply take a moment of mindfulness every day and self-love unfolds...

# Hypnosis 7

## Goal Setting and Preparation

You want to be able to accept yourself... more than that, you want to love yourself... Self-love is like a warm feeling from you for you... a warm feeling from you for you... You know the feeling of love... it is a feeling of warmth... like the warmth of a very intimate embrace... So is self-love, because it is like an inner self-embrace... Your body can help you to experience such an embrace inside... deep within your inner center, you can embrace yourself... maybe initially as an imagination or a wish... and then also as a real feeling... because everything you can imagine can also become truth in your feeling... Your body can help you with this... Maybe you are already curiously wondering how exactly it works that your body helps you with an inner embrace... Your body can give you signals... It does so constantly... Our bodies are constantly talking to us, we just have to listen... and listening means feeling in the body... So find a place in your body that feels warm... maybe just a little warmer than another place... maybe on your back or in your belly... maybe you also feel warmth in your feet or hands... Never do all parts of the body feel the same... There are always areas, places or zones that are somewhat cooler... others are a bit warmer and more pleasant... So you can quickly find the warmest spot on your body... and imagine that exactly there, where the warmest spot on your body is, also lies the potential for your self-love... wherever that spot may be... Indeed, the possibility of unfolding warmth and letting it work for the whole body lies in the warm areas of the body... Maybe you think it has to do with your clothing, the blanket or the room temperature, which place on your body simply feels warmer... but your body knows it can direct your attention... can make you aware of a warm spot... and while you focus entirely on this spot, your body sends all your potential for self-acceptance and self-love exactly there to show you something... So you can trust your body to help you... You now find a pleasant and warm spot... You find it on your body... go entirely there, with all your mindfulness and attention... Focus on this warmth...

Somato-emotional Change

Now your body feeling helps you... Maybe the spot you found is indeed only coincidentally warmer than another, but that does not matter... Your body can do something special... It can communicate with you, can send you messages... Now keep your concentration on the spot you found, wherever it is... It can remain your secret... Your subconscious now bundles your potential for affection and love... your potential for self-love... because just as you can feel affection for others, so you can feel affection for yourself... Your subconscious bundles this power and sends it to the warm spot you found... and the more you manage to focus your attention on this spot and concentrate, the more potential your subconscious, your deep inner self can also send there... and the spot becomes even warmer... This is how your body tells you that it is indeed working... that really at this moment your own potential is being sent there and is now arriving there... The pleasant spot becomes warmer... very pleasantly warm... You only need to focus on it... That is enough... You have this potential for love within you, because you manage to feel affection and love for others... You also have this potential for affection for yourself and the potential for self-love, because it is the same potential... but today just for you... today only for you... You feel the warmth now more clearly... the more you manage to focus entirely on the warm zone, the more pleasantly warm it becomes... it succeeds for you... Excellent, how well it already succeeds for you... Now feel this beautiful warmth very precisely... perceive it intensely, because it is warmth within you... warmth from you for you... warmth only from you... only for you... your self-warmth... your self-love... which now may unfold...

And as a sign that your self-love may now fully unfold and spread within you... this warmth feeling spreads throughout your whole body... Imagine the warmth like a sun shining within you... like the warming light of a beautiful candle spreading out... then you feel how from the warm zone warmth slowly and evenly radiates through your entire body... then you feel how your inner warmth now spreads slowly and flows through your whole body, becoming warmer... It is as if the temperature in the room is increased and everything around you becomes warmer... everything inside you becomes warmer... Your body shows you with this that your potential is indeed unfolding within you... as a sign... as a signal from your body that you are now truly ready to accept yourself... that you are now truly ready to let your self-warmth work for you... warmth from you for you... love from you for you... A warm feeling spreads within you and you can feel it now when you pay attention to your body and feel... This is your warmth... This is your self-love...

### Reinforcement (Posthypnotic Suggestion)

Isn't it wonderful how well you can feel it... how easily your body can show and prove to you that it works for you to love yourself... Whenever you want to reassure yourself that it always works for you to love yourself, you can find the warmth in your body in a state of calm and feel how it spreads... just like today... exactly like today...

# Hypnosis 8

### Ideomotoric

*Ideomotorics refers to the phenomenon that our body follows our feelings and thoughts with movements. In everyday life, this following shows as body posture, muscle tension, and movement patterns of a person, which naturally change with the mood and thoughts. In trance, ideomotoric signals can be used to obtain information that the client cannot actively communicate. For example, the subconscious can answer questions with an agreed finger signal. Of course, ideomotoric reactions can also be used suggestively, for example, with arm levitations and catalepsies. An ideomotoric approach strengthens trust in hypnosis and one's ability to change, thus promoting therapy.*

### Setting Up Finger Signals

Dear subconscious of [Client's Name], with the index finger, you greeted me and showed your willingness to cooperate... thank you for that... The index finger will therefore stand for the answer YES... whenever you want to say YES, you can move the index finger clearly, let's try it... if you understand me, move the index finger of your right hand... [Wait until the finger moves]... very good... but it can also be that you want to say NO, so we need a finger for the answer NO... We take the little finger for this... Now move the little finger for the answer NO... Move the little finger as a sign of the answer NO... [Wait until the finger moves]... Thank you very much! So, we take the index finger for YES and the little finger for NO... It can begin...

Choosing a Suitable Role Model

You don't always manage to love and appreciate yourself because you mostly take care of the well-being of others first... but you know people who do it differently... who manage to accept and appreciate themselves... to love themselves... They can do it, and it looks easy when they do it... It is quite natural for them to love themselves... You wish for it too, and sometimes you thought it would be nice if you could do it too... perhaps you wondered how they do it... Your subconscious knows how they do it and why they succeed... You don't need to strain your mind; you can leave the work to your subconscious... Subconscious of [Client's

Name], consider the people who manage to accept and love themselves... You know they are not more lovable or different, you know they just take a different attitude towards themselves... an attitude you can also adopt... Choose, subconscious of [Client's Name], from the many role models you know inside, the role model that can do it best, the person who succeeds best in truly accepting and loving themselves, just as you want to... and as soon as you have found this role model, show me with the YES finger... Show me the YES finger as soon as you have found the best role model... [Wait until the finger moves]... Thank you, you have found the right role model...

Learning from the Role Model

Now see for yourself, just for you and deep within you, how this person manages it... what they do differently and better to accept themselves as they are... and learn from this role model how to do it... You can do it and you will manage it... Watch closely how this person treats themselves to love themselves... Is this what you need as well? [Wait for the finger signal, if YES, continue reading, if NO, first let them find a new role model]... It is the right role model, very good! Now feel into your role model to learn from them... feel and understand how your role model treats themselves and learn... and you, subconscious of [Client's Name], can learn faster than the mind... Feel the positive thoughts of self-love of your role model... Feel the body movements of your role model that enhance the feeling of self-love... recognize the pattern of self-perception and self-love of your role model, which can become your own pattern... Learn, subconscious of [Client's Name], just for you and in silence, how your role model manages to be good to themselves, to love themselves... because you can do it too... Make this strength of your role model your own... make it your own strength and your success... because you too can accept and love yourself... You are now learning from your role model how it works... You learn without having to think... you learn without having to think... You learn in feeling because you recognize the feeling of your role model... Adopt the best from your role model because you may learn from them today, may simply copy their ability and naturalness to accept and love themselves and make it your own feeling and action... your action towards yourself so that you can accept and love yourself just as your role model does... and as soon as you have succeeded in this learning, show me the YES finger... Answer with the YES finger as soon as you have deeply learned to accept and love yourself... This learning, this change is happening right now deep inside you and is very simple... Your YES finger will soon show that it has indeed succeeded... [Wait until the YES finger moves; don't worry, it will happen if you remain calm and don't pressure]... You have succeeded! Well done, you have indeed succeeded... now you manage to accept and love yourself just as your role model does...

Resolving the Ideomotoric Signals

You have accomplished a lot and now everything will be different... Thank you, dear subconscious of [Client's Name]... You can now release the control of the right hand and spread out in the whole body... As soon as you wake up again and arrive in your everyday life, you will feel that you have indeed succeeded in loving yourself better... much more than before... You can now let go of all images and fantasies inside and feel comfortable in your whole body... Allow yourself calm and serenity and trust that today you have learned from your role model how to fully accept yourself, how to fully love yourself...

[Please try to be patient if the signals come hesitantly. Ideomotoric signals are reliable signs, similar to kinesiological muscle tests. The brief reframing presented here is very effective in practice when ideomotoric signals are given as confirmation. If communicating with finger signals is difficult, deepen the trance in between with simple suggestions. More detailed work with reframings can be found in my book "Reframing in Trance".]

# Hypnosis 9

### Arriving in the Land of Dreams

Fantasy and reality sometimes seem like two worlds... but sometimes they are very close together... Then fantasy can become reality or already be reality... and often we cannot even distinguish what is real and what is thought... what already exists or what is still a wish that may soon become reality... There is a land deep inside you where you can find all this... fantasy and reality... a land where you can build a bridge between what is still fantasy today and what may become reality tomorrow... your reality... the reality of your feelings... It is the land of dreams... Your wishes bring you there... You are already there... deep in your fantasy, where your feelings can become images... You are in the land of dreams... like in another time... in another world... and yet very close to you... closer perhaps than ever before...

### Colors and Healing in the Dreamland

[gray]... You are standing high up on a mountain, far north, and you see a snow-covered landscape... mountains

and valleys, meadows and forests, covered in snow... You are warmly wrapped and feel good, looking at the evening sky... There you see colorful lights, you see the northern lights changing colors... and each color reminds you of something from your life... The sky glows gray and reminds you of the hard times in your life... often it could not succeed for you to bear yourself because you blamed yourself for everything... because you thought everything that went wrong was your fault... then you often rejected yourself... but kept going and tried to make the best of it... [White]... Then you look into the valley and over the land and see the sparkling white snow... It shines so brightly that the gray of the sky can no longer bother you... The white sparkle reminds you that there were always bright spots in life and still are... that you also succeeded again and again in being more reconciled with yourself and being able to bear yourself well... perhaps there were even white times or at least white moments when you liked or loved yourself... The white shining snow reminds you that it can succeed again... [light blue]... Then you direct your gaze back up to the evening sky and see a light blue northern light spreading quickly and overstraining the whole sky... The color light blue shows you in the land of dreams that the endless expanse of life is open to you again once you manage to lovingly let go of the past because you cannot change the past anymore... if you could not accept yourself in the past, you cannot do it retroactively... but you can look forward and this look is light blue... [golden yellow]... Then the sky glows in a strong golden yellow, as beautiful as sunflowers... Golden yellow is the color of learning, recognizing, and understanding... It reminds you that you had to learn many things in life... some painfully and difficult, others also easily and lightly... In the land of dreams, the color golden yellow helps you to learn quite easily how to do it... to like yourself again and to be one with yourself... [red]... Then the color of the northern lights changes and you see a red glow filling the sky more and more... Red, you certainly know as the color of love... Red is also the color of self-love... The red glow reminds you that it is a wish to be able to love yourself... In the land of dreams and fantasies, only what can also exist in reality exists... because everything here is feeling... every image, every color is a feeling... and red is the feeling of self-love... the love from you for you that shines here for you... even if you cannot feel it yet or only a little, this red glow shows you that it is there and always will be... [silver]... Then you see a thousand little stars in the sky, shining and sparkling silver for you, and the North Star shines especially brightly for you... It looks like it is made of pure silver... Silver is in the land of dreams the color of a good future... the color of the beautiful and coming reality that may be as soon as the right time has come... and maybe this time is just now, in this moment and the silver glow helps you now to accept yourself better and maybe even feel a bit of self-love already... now in this moment, who knows... [gold]... Then the sky sparkles golden... and golden light spreads out... the light of creation... the light of life force... the deep life force within you... You see this golden glow, the most beautiful light you have ever seen... it shows you that there is a great and indestructible power within you... a power with which you can achieve anything... a power that helps you to love yourself... to love yourself fully and completely...

Mindfulness and Self-loyalty

Then you look over the landscape before you... You can look endlessly far into the distance, see houses and villages in the snow-covered landscape... You see the wide valleys and beautiful forests... the most beautiful land you have ever seen, bathed in beautiful white snow... in the shining white color... in the shining white light... The land of dreams is open to you... the land of your dreams, where you can achieve anything... and everything you can achieve, you can also achieve in your feeling... Self-love... love from you for you... It succeeds because the land of dreams is not just a fantasy... the land of dreams is reality... It lies deep within you... It has always been there... I am just telling you about it...

# Hypnosis 10

### Arriving in the Land of Dreams

Fantasy and reality sometimes seem like two worlds... but sometimes they are very close together... Then fantasy can become reality or already be reality... and often we cannot even distinguish what is real and what is thought... what already exists or what is still a wish that may soon become reality... There is a land deep inside you where you can find all this... fantasy and reality... a land where you can build a bridge between what is still fantasy today and what may become reality tomorrow... your reality... the reality of your feelings... It is the land of dreams... Your wishes bring you there... You are already there... deep in your fantasy, where your feelings can become images... You are in the land of dreams... like in another time... in another world... and yet very close to you... closer perhaps than ever before...

### Confrontation, Clarification, and Creative Reorientation

You are standing on a beautiful flower meadow... the weather is just as you like it best, because in the land of dreams everything follows your wish and your feeling... maybe the sun should shine in a beautiful golden yellow color... or you prefer a sky full of white clouds... or both together... You can decide for yourself... Then you start walking, step by step... you don't need a goal or direction in the land of dreams because you cannot get lost here, cannot go astray... Every step in the land of dreams is a step towards yourself... every path always leads only to you... So walk at your own pace towards yourself... in your own tempo... Time does not matter here, because it does not exist... Everything happens in the moment and time is only the illusion of memory... You find a nice place to rest... to rest from the exertions and strains of life... from laborious experiences and painful memories... maybe in the shade of a tree or in the sun... There can be a mattress or a hammock between trees... or you just lie down in the meadow... on the ground, in the grass... just as you wish... You close your eyes and start to dream... In dream images, you see again experiences that led you to reject yourself... or to barely bear yourself... You see yourself as a stranger because you often felt alien to yourself and within yourself... often felt little closeness to yourself... maybe you also sometimes forbade yourself to accept and like yourself... thought it was not right to really like yourself... to embrace yourself inwardly and to love yourself...

Then you hear children's voices in the wind and you open your eyes to see where the voices are coming from... Children's voices in the land of dreams... Then you see a group of children running across the meadow, coming straight towards you... They wave and call your name because they know you... perhaps better than you know yourself... You wonder who they might be and where they come from... and one of these children looks familiar... You have seen this face often because it is your child's face... The child looks like you... but all of them look familiar... They greet you and sit down with you to tell you stories... They tell you about their lives... The child that looks like you as a child tells you that it cannot love itself... It is forbidden, it says... it has learned to care more about others... it has learned to neglect itself... and this child also tells you how that came to be... You listen to its words and hear your own story... The child tells of you... because it is you yourself who tells this in the land of dreams... Then other children also tell that they cannot love themselves, but it is their special wish... and in each child, you recognize something of yourself because they all resemble you... one wears the shoes you wore as a child... another wears clothes from your childhood... and another child has your childhood hairstyle... So each of these children resembles you in their own way and each tells you a part of your story... and all seek affection and love in the land of dreams... Affection and love in the land of dreams can only ever be self-love... You take the children in your arms, embrace each of them and rest with them together... and all look together into the light blue sky... and memories pass by like small white clouds in the sky... driven by the wind... and no one can hold them in the land of dreams... Memories go with the wind and the sky becomes light blue again... The children jump up and want to run on... Each gives you a red rose as a sign of affection and connection... and the child that looks most like you, that looks just as you did as a child, gives you the biggest and most beautiful red rose... Then they say goodbye and with new strength and joy they run towards the horizon... at the horizon, the future begins... and the future begins already in the next moment...

Mindfulness and Self-loyalty

You watch the children leave... your smile accompanies them to the horizon... You think about the fact that it is the memories that have held you back for so long... have prevented you for so long from loving yourself... Here in the land of dreams, the children manage to accept you and give you a sign of love... You look at the red roses and it becomes clear to you that each child is a part of yourself... so it is you who can accept and give yourself a gift of love here... love from you for you... in the land of dreams, it is possible, but what is possible here can succeed anywhere... also and especially in your waking everyday life... You realize again that the land of dreams lies deep within you... it has always been there... I am just telling you about it...

Distribution, publication, and copying in any form are prohibited and subject to damages.

## Overview of All Titles in the Series "Ten Hypnoses"

Volume 1: Smoking Cessation
Volume 2: Anxiety and Restlessness
Volume 3: Burnout
Volume 4: Reducing Overweight
Volume 5: Coping with the Past
Volume 6: Suicidal Thoughts and Attempts
Volume 7: Psycho-Oncology
Volume 8: Obsessions and Tics
Volume 9: Self-Confidence and Decision-Making
Volume 10: Grief Work
Volume 11: Psychosomatics
Volume 12: Chronic Pain
Volume 13: Depressive Thoughts
Volume 14: Panic Attacks
Volume 15: Domestic Violence, Victim Support
Volume 16: Post-Traumatic Stress
Volume 17: Exam Anxiety and Stage Fright
Volume 18: Anti-Violence Training, Offender Support
Volume 19: Addiction Tendencies
Volume 20: Social Phobia and Fear of Contact
Volume 21: Nail Biting
Volume 22: Self-Awareness and Self-Love
Volume 23: Teeth Grinding and Night Clenching
Volume 24: Feelings of Guilt
Volume 25: Fear in Crowds
Volume 26: Fear of Flying, Aviophobia
Volume 27: Fear in Enclosed Spaces, Claustrophobia
Volume 28: Tinnitus, Ear Noises
Volume 29: Fear of Heights
Volume 30: Neurodermatitis

Copying, publishing, and sharing with third parties are only permitted with the written consent of the author. Please observe the notes on copyright and usage.

Volume 31: Finding Inner Balance
Volume 32: Overcoming Loneliness
Volume 33: Fear of Illness, Hypochondria
Volume 34: Anticipatory Anxiety, Fear of Fear
Volume 35: Jealousy in Relationships
Volume 36: Driving Anxiety
Volume 37: New Start after Separation
Volume 38: Fear of Injections
Volume 39: Heart Anxiety Neurosis
Volume 40: Overcoming Resentment and Anger
Volume 41: Resolving Blockages and Positive Thinking
Volume 42: Stress Reduction, Stress Management
Volume 43: Body Relaxation
Volume 44: Deep Relaxation
Volume 45: Fear of the Dark
Volume 46: Falling Asleep and Staying Asleep
Volume 47: Compulsive Buying
Volume 48: Restless Legs Syndrome
Volume 49: Bulimia
Volume 50: Anorexia
Volume 51: Overcoming Nightmares
Volume 52: Imagined Deformity
Volume 53: Overcoming Distrust, Finding Trust
Volume 54: Processing Failures
Volume 55: Humiliation, Emotional Hurt
Volume 56: Distressing Compassion, Vicarious Suffering
Volume 57: Self-Forgiveness
Volume 58: Self-Awareness, Self-Confidence
Volume 59: Saying No
Volume 60: Assertiveness
Volume 61: Setting Boundaries and Self-Assertion
Volume 62: Decision-Making Ability

Volume 63: Success Orientation
Volume 64: Ruminating, Circular Thinking
Volume 65: Accepting Pregnancy
Volume 66: Birth Preparation
Volume 67: Spiritual Opening
Volume 68: Joy of Life and Inner Lightness
Volume 69: Patience and Inner Peace
Volume 70: Fibromyalgia and Rheumatism
Volume 71: Irritable Bowel Syndrome, Crohn's Disease
Volume 72: Fear of Nausea, Emetophobia
Volume 73: Stuttering and Cluttering, Speech Flow Disorders
Volume 74: Concentration and Knowledge Anchoring
Volume 75: Vitality and Spontaneity
Volume 76: Searching for Meaning and Finding Goals
Volume 77: Life Crises, Life Events
Volume 78: Workaholism, Goal Obsession
Volume 79: Helper Syndrome, Helpless Helpers
Volume 80: Medication Abuse
Volume 81: Gambling Addiction
Volume 82: Internet Addiction, Smartphone Addiction
Volume 83: Hoarding Disorder, Compulsive Collecting
Volume 84: Conspiracy Thoughts, Overvalued Ideas
Volume 85: Fear of Operations and Treatments
Volume 86: Fear of Aging
Volume 87: Travel Anxiety
Volume 88: Anxiety When Urinating, Paruresis
Volume 89: Fear of Intimacy and Togetherness
Volume 90: Fear of Blushing
Volume 91: Coming Out in Homosexuality
Volume 92: Charisma Training
Volume 93: Migraines and Chronic Headaches
Volume 94: Overcoming Allergies, Bronchial Asthma

Volume 95: Normalizing Blood Pressure
Volume 96: Compulsive Perfectionism
Volume 97: Sports Hypnosis, Motivation
Volume 98: Sports Hypnosis, Performance Enhancement
Volume 99: Determination and Focus
Volume 100: Encountering the Inner Child
Volume 101: Cravings, Binge Eating
Volume 102: Stimulating Metabolism
Volume 103: Bipolar Mood Swings
Volume 104: Borderline, Identity Crises
Volume 105: Hypomania, Euphoria, Mania
Volume 106: Restlessness, Agitation
Volume 107: Nervous Breakdown
Volume 108: Adjustment Disorders
Volume 109: Self-Alienation, Depersonalization
Volume 110: Ending Self-Pity
Volume 111: Primary Gain of Illness
Volume 112: Secondary Gain of Illness
Volume 113: Bullying, Victim Support
Volume 114: Letting Go of Envy and Jealousy
Volume 115: Fear of Spiders, Arachnophobia
Volume 116: Fear of Dogs or Cats
Volume 117: Fear of Strangers, Xenophobia
Volume 118: Excessive Worries, Generalized Anxiety
Volume 119: Strengthening Sense of Responsibility
Volume 120: Unrequited Love, Heartache
Volume 121: Work-Life Balance
Volume 122: Letting Go of Unattainable Goals
Volume 123: Allowing and Accepting Help
Volume 124: Letting Go of Adult Children
Volume 125: Tourette Syndrome
Volume 126: Life Changes and New Starts

Volume 127: Accepting Life in a Wheelchair
Volume 128: Understanding and Overcoming Homesickness
Volume 129: Understanding and Overcoming Wanderlust
Volume 130: Dizziness, Meniere's Disease
Volume 131: Overcoming Aggression
Volume 132: Cutting and Self-Harm
Volume 133: Hair Pulling, Trichotillomania
Volume 134: Postpartum Depression
Volume 135: For Relatives of Dementia Patients
Volume 136: Self-Harm, Artificial Disorders
Volume 137: Activating Self-Healing Powers
Volume 138: Preventing Depression Relapse
Volume 139: Reactive Psychoses, Follow-Up
Volume 140: Obsessive Thoughts and Impulses
Volume 141: Compulsive Checking
Volume 142: Compulsive Counting, Symmetry Obsession
Volume 143: Compulsive Washing, Cleanliness Obsession
Volume 144: Compulsive Questioning
Volume 145: Dissociative Paralysis
Volume 146: Phantom Pain
Volume 147: Overcoming Complaining
Volume 148: Hay Fever, Pollen Allergy
Volume 149: Sexual Abuse, Victim Support
Volume 150: Standing Strong Against Sexism, #metoo
Volume 151: Binge Eating
Volume 152: Overcoming Thoughts of Revenge
Volume 153: Detachment from the Aggressor, Stockholm Syndrome
Volume 154: Courage to Separate
Volume 155: Chronic Fatigue, Exhaustion
Volume 156: Fear of the Future, Existential Anxiety
Volume 157: Excessive Worry About Children
Volume 158: Fear of Failure

Volume 159: Ending Distrust and Control
Volume 160: Dejection, Dysphoria
Volume 161: Boreout, Chronic Boredom
Volume 162: Bipolar Disorders, Relapse Prevention
Volume 163: Mania, Relapse Prevention
Volume 164: Nihilism, Feelings of Worthlessness
Volume 165: Thumb Sucking
Volume 166: Being Brave
Volume 167: Being Proud
Volume 168: Overcoming Shyness
Volume 169: Being Able to Delegate Responsibility
Volume 170: Being Able to Show Emotions
Volume 171: Letting Go of Guilt, Victim Support
Volume 172: Processing Guilt, Offender Support
Volume 173: Mood Swings, Cyclothymia
Volume 174: Lack of Drive, Vital Sadness
Volume 175: Hearing Voices with Reality Reference
Volume 176: Confident Communication
Volume 177: Standing Up for Oneself
Volume 178: Taking New Paths
Volume 179: Confident Job Application
Volume 180: No Longer Being Taken Advantage Of
Volume 181: End of Submissiveness
Volume 182: Depressive Numbness
Volume 183: Mood Drops, Affective Incontinence
Volume 184: Mood Instability
Volume 185: Somatoform Disorders
Volume 186: Stomach Ulcer, Psychosomatic
Volume 187: Accepting Amputation
Volume 188: Overcoming and Letting Go of Hatred
Volume 189: Ending Accusations
Volume 190: Allowing Tears, Being Able to Cry

Volume 191: Finding and Sorting Repressed Feelings
Volume 192: Somatoform Pain
Volume 193: Living Autonomously
Volume 194: Anhedonia, Joylessness
Volume 195: Persistent Sadness
Volume 196: Obesity, Food Addiction
Volume 197: Parents of Abused Children
Volume 198: Letting Go and Letting Be
Volume 199: Childhood Sexual Abuse
Volume 200: Fear of Loss

www.ingramcontent.com/pod-product-compliance
Lightning Source LLC
Chambersburg PA
CBHW030501220526
45464CB00006B/2602